The Easiest

CW00376735

Cookbook

Simple, Quick and Easy Dash Diet Recipes

Candace Hickman

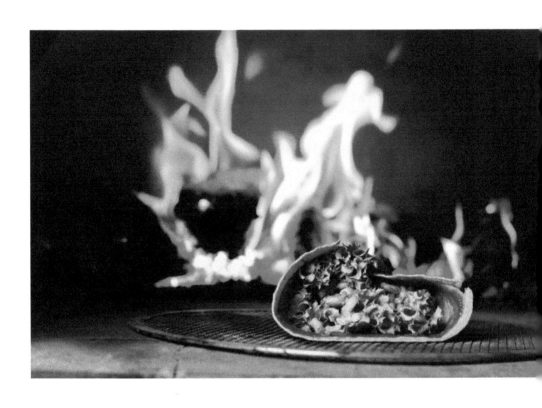

© Copyright 2021 - All rights reserved.

The content contained within this book may not be reproduced, duplicated or transmitted without direct written permission from the author or the publisher.

Under no circumstances will any blame or legal responsibility be held against the publisher, or author, for any damages, reparation, or monetary loss due to the information contained within this book. Either directly or indirectly.

Legal Notice:

This book is copyright protected. This book is only for personal use. You cannot amend, distribute, sell, use, quote or paraphrase any part, or the content within this book, without the consent of the author or publisher.

Disclaimer Notice:

Please note the information contained within this document is for educational and entertainment purposes only. All effort has been executed to present accurate, up to date, and reliable, complete information. No warranties of any kind are declared or implied. Readers acknowledge that the author is not engaging in the rendering of legal, financial, medical or professional advice. The content within this book has been derived from various sources. Please consult a licensed professional before attempting any techniques outlined in this book.

By reading this document, the reader agrees that under no circumstances is the author responsible for any losses, direct or indirect, which are incurred as a result of the use of information contained within this document, including, but not limited to, — errors, omissions, or inaccuracies.

TABLE OF CONTENT

Mushroom Salad

Preparation time: 10 minutes

Cooking time: 20 minutes

Servings: 4

Ingredients:

- 10 ounces smoked salmon, low-sodium, boneless, skinless and cubed
- 2 green onions, chopped
- 2 red chili peppers, chopped
- 1 tablespoon olive oil
- ½ teaspoon oregano, dried
- ½ teaspoon smoked paprika
- A pinch of black pepper
- 8 ounces white mushrooms, sliced
- 1 tablespoon lemon juice
- 1 cup black olives, pitted and halved
- 1 tablespoon parsley, chopped

Directions:

1. Heat up a pan with the oil over medium heat, add the onions and chili peppers, stir and cook for 4 minutes.

2. Add the mushrooms, stir and sauté them for 5 minutes.
3. Add the salmon and the other ingredients, toss, cook everything for 10 minutes more, divide into bowls and serve for lunch.

Nutrition info per serving: 95 calories, 3.7g protein, 5.1g carbohydrates, 7.7g fat, 2.2g fiber, 2mg cholesterol, 355mg sodium, 240mg potassium

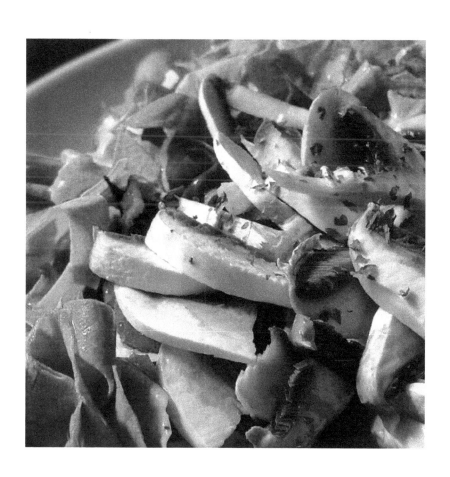

Chickpeas Pan

Preparation time: 10 minutes

Cooking time: 30 minutes

Servings: 4

Ingredients:

- 2 tablespoons olive oil
- 1 cup canned chickpeas, no-salt-added, drained and rinsed
- 1 pound sweet potatoes, peeled and cut into wedges
- 4 garlic cloves, minced
- 2 shallots, chopped
- 1 cup canned tomatoes, no-salt-added and chopped
- 1 teaspoon coriander, ground
- 2 tomatoes, chopped
- 1 cup low-sodium vegetable stock
- A pinch of black pepper
- 1 tablespoon lemon juice
- 1 tablespoon cilantro, chopped

Directions:

1. Heat up a pot with the oil over medium heat, add the shallots and the garlic, stir and sauté for 5 minutes.
2. Add the chickpeas, potatoes and the other ingredients, bring to a simmer and cook over medium heat for 25 minutes.
3. Divide everything into bowls and serve for lunch.

Nutrition info per serving: 450 calories, 15g protein, 78.5g carbohydrates, 10.7g fat, 16.7g fiber, 0mg cholesterol, 126mg sodium, 2169mg potassium

Turmeric Chicken Mix

Preparation time: 10 minutes

Cooking time: 30 minutes

Servings: 4

Ingredients:

- 1 tablespoon olive oil
- 1 pound chicken breast, skinless, boneless and cubed
- 1 shallot, chopped
- 1 tablespoon ginger, grated
- 2 garlic cloves, minced
- 1 teaspoon cardamom, ground
- ½ teaspoon turmeric powder
- 1 teaspoon lime juice
- 1 cup low-sodium chicken stock
- 1 tablespoon cilantro, chopped

Directions:

1. Heat up a pot with the oil over medium-high heat, add the shallot, ginger, garlic, cardamom and the turmeric, stir and sauté for 5 minutes.
2. Add the meat and brown it for 5 minutes.

3. Add the rest of the ingredients, bring everything to a simmer and cook for 20 minutes.
4. Divide the mix into bowls and serve.

Nutrition info per serving: 176 calories, 25g protein, 3.1g carbohydrates, 6.5g fat, 0.4g fiber, 73mg cholesterol, 77mg sodium, 474mg potassium

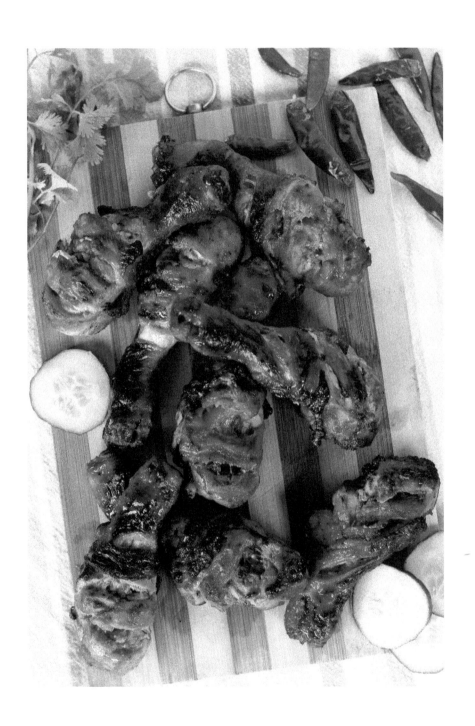

Chipotle Lentils

Preparation time: 10 minutes

Cooking time: 35 minutes

Servings: 6

Ingredients:

- 1 green bell pepper, chopped
- 1 tablespoon olive oil
- 2 spring onions, chopped
- 2 garlic cloves, minced
- 24 ounces canned lentils, no-salt-added, drained and rinsed
- 2 cups veggie stock
- 2 tablespoons chili powder, mild
- ½ teaspoon chipotle powder
- 30 ounces canned tomatoes, no-salt-added, chopped
- A pinch of black pepper

Directions:

1. Heat up a pot with the oil over medium heat, add the onions and the garlic, stir and sauté for 5 minutes.

2. Add the bell pepper, lentils and the other ingredients, bring to a simmer and cook over medium heat for 30 minutes.
3. Divide the chili into bowls and serve for lunch.

Nutrition info per serving: 476 calories, 32.8g protein, 77.5g carbohydrates, 4.8g fat, 37.6g fiber, 0mg cholesterol, 295mg sodium, 1591mg potassium

Turmeric Endives

Preparation time: 10 minutes

Cooking time: 20 minutes

Servings: 4

Ingredients:

- 2 endives, halved lengthwise
- 2 tablespoons olive oil
- 1 teaspoon rosemary, dried
- ½ teaspoon turmeric powder
- A pinch of black pepper

Directions:

1. In a baking pan, combine the endives with the oil and the other ingredients, toss gently, introduce in the oven and bake at 400 degrees F for 20 minutes.
2. Divide between plates and serve as a side dish.

Nutrition info per serving: 64 calories, 0.2g protein, 0.8g carbohydrates, 7.1g fat, 0.6g fiber, 0mg cholesterol, 3mg sodium, 50mg potassium

Parmesan Endives

Preparation time: 10 minutes

Cooking time: 20 minutes

Servings: 4

Ingredients:

- 4 endives, halved lengthwise
- 1 tablespoon lemon juice
- 1 tablespoon lemon zest, grated
- 2 tablespoons fat-free parmesan, grated
- 2 tablespoons olive oil
- A pinch of black pepper

Directions:

1. In a baking dish, combine the endives with the lemon juice and the other ingredients except the parmesan and toss.
2. Sprinkle the parmesan on top, bake the endives at 400 degrees F for 20 minutes, divide between plates and serve as a side dish.

Nutrition info per serving: 71 calories, 0.9g protein, 2.2g carbohydrates, 7.1g fat, 0.9g fiber, 0mg cholesterol, 71mg sodium, 88mg potassium

Lemon Asparagus

Preparation time: 10 minutes

Cooking time: 20 minutes

Servings: 4

Ingredients:

- 1 pound asparagus, trimmed
- 2 tablespoons basil pesto
- 1 tablespoon lemon juice
- A pinch of black pepper
- 3 tablespoons olive oil
- 2 tablespoons cilantro, chopped

Directions:

1. Arrange the asparagus n a lined baking sheet, add the pesto and the other ingredients, toss, introduce in the oven and cook at 400 degrees F for 20 minutes.
2. Divide between plates and serve as a side dish.

Nutrition info per serving: 114 calories, 2.6g protein, 4.5g carbohydrates, 10.7g fat, 2.4g fiber, 0mg cholesterol, 3mg sodium, 240mg potassium

Lime Carrots

Preparation time: 10 minutes

Cooking time: 30 minutes

Servings: 4

Ingredients:

- 1 pound baby carrots, trimmed
- 1 tablespoon sweet paprika
- 1 teaspoon lime juice
- 3 tablespoons olive oil
- A pinch of black pepper
- 1 teaspoon sesame seeds

Directions:

1. Arrange the carrots on a lined baking sheet, add the paprika and the other ingredients except the sesame seeds, toss, introduce in the oven and bake at 400 degrees F for 30 minutes.
2. Divide the carrots between plates, sprinkle sesame seeds on top and serve as a side dish.

Nutrition info per serving: 139 calories, 1.1g protein, 10.5g carbohydrates, 11.2g fat, 4g fiber, 0mg cholesterol, 89mg sodium, 313mg potassium

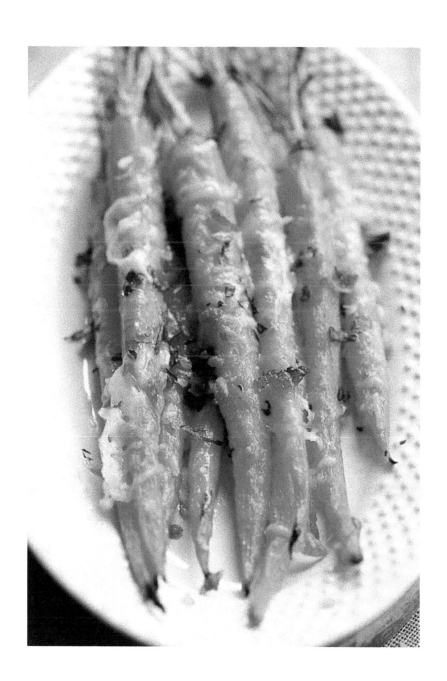

Garlic Potato Pan

Preparation time: 10 minutes

Cooking time: 1 hour

Servings: 8

Ingredients:

- 1 pound gold potatoes, peeled and cut into wedges
- 2 tablespoons olive oil
- 1 red onion, chopped
- 2 garlic cloves, minced
- 2 cups coconut cream
- 1 tablespoon thyme, chopped
- ¼ teaspoon nutmeg, ground
- ½ cup low-fat parmesan, grated

Directions:

1. Heat up a pan with the oil over medium heat, add the onion and the garlic and sauté for 5 minutes.
2. Add the potatoes and brown them for 5 minutes more.
3. Add the cream and the rest of the ingredients, toss gently, bring to a simmer

and cook over medium heat for 40 minutes more.

4. Divide the mix between plates and serve as a side dish.

Nutrition info per serving: 230 calories, 3.6g protein, 14.3g carbohydrates, 19.1g fat, 3.3g fiber, 6mg cholesterol, 105mg sodium, 426mg potassium

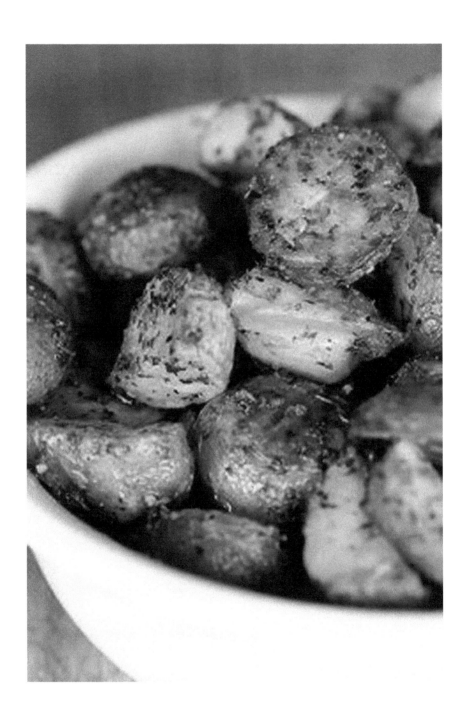

Balsamic Cabbage

Preparation time: 10 minutes

Cooking time: 20 minutes

Servings: 4

Ingredients:

- 1 pound green cabbage, roughly shredded
- 2 tablespoons olive oil
- A pinch of black pepper
- 1 shallot, chopped
- 2 garlic cloves, minced
- 2 tablespoons balsamic vinegar
- 2 teaspoons hot paprika
- 1 teaspoon sesame seeds

Directions:

1. Heat up a pan with the oil over medium heat, add the shallot and the garlic and sauté for 5 minutes.
2. Add the cabbage and the other ingredients, toss, cook over medium heat for 15 minutes, divide between plates and serve.

Nutrition info per serving: 100 calories, 1.8g protein, 8.2g carbohydrates, 7.5g fat, 3g fiber, 0mg cholesterol, 22mg sodium, 225mg potassium

Chili Broccoli

Preparation time: 10 minutes

Cooking time: 30 minutes

Servings: 4

Ingredients:

- 2 tablespoons olive oil
- 1 pound broccoli florets
- 2 garlic cloves, minced
- 2 tablespoons chili sauce
- 1 tablespoon lemon juice
- A pinch of black pepper
- 2 tablespoons cilantro, chopped

Directions:

1. In a baking pan, combine the broccoli with the oil, garlic and the other ingredients, toss a bit, introduce in the oven and bake at 400 degrees F for 30 minutes.
2. Divide the mix between plates and serve as a side dish.

Nutrition info per serving: 103 calories, 3.4g protein, 8.3g carbohydrates, 7.4g fat, 3g fiber, 0mg cholesterol, 229mg sodium, 383mg potassium

Hot Brussels Sprouts

Preparation time: 10 minutes

Cooking time: 25 minutes

Servings: 4

Ingredients:

- 1 tablespoon olive oil
- 1 pound Brussels sprouts, trimmed and halved
- 2 garlic cloves, minced
- ½ cup low-fat mozzarella, shredded
- A pinch of pepper flakes, crushed

Directions:

1. In a baking dish, combine the sprouts with the oil and the other ingredients except the cheese and toss.
2. Sprinkle the cheese on top, introduce in the oven and bake at 400 degrees F for 25 minutes.
3. Divide between plates and serve as a side dish.

Nutrition info per serving: 111 calories, 10g protein, 11.6g carbohydrates, 3.9g fat, 5g fiber, 4mg cholesterol, 209mg sodium, 447mg potassium

Paprika Brussels Sprouts

Preparation time: 10 minutes

Cooking time: 25 minutes

Servings: 4

Ingredients:

- 2 tablespoons olive oil
- 1 pound Brussels sprouts, trimmed and halved
- 3 green onions, chopped
- 2 garlic cloves, minced
- 1 tablespoon balsamic vinegar
- 1 tablespoon sweet paprika
- A pinch of black pepper

Directions:

1. In a baking pan, combine the Brussels sprouts with the oil and the other ingredients, toss and bake at 400 degrees F for 25 minutes.
2. Divide the mix between plates and serve.

Nutrition info per serving: 121 calories, 4.4g protein, 12.6g carbohydrates, 7.6g fat, 5.2g fiber, 0mg cholesterol, 31mg sodium, 521mg potassium

Creamy Cauliflower Mash

Preparation time: 10 minutes

Cooking time: 25 minutes

Servings: 4

Ingredients:

- 2 pounds cauliflower florets
- ½ cup coconut milk
- A pinch of black pepper
- ½ cup low-fat sour cream
- 1 tablespoon cilantro, chopped
- 1 tablespoon chives, chopped

Directions:

1. Put the cauliflower in a pot, add water to cover, bring to a boil over medium heat, cook for 25 minutes and drain.
2. Mash the cauliflower, add the milk, black pepper and the cream, whisk well, divide between plates, sprinkle the rest of the ingredients on top and serve.

Nutrition info per serving: 188 calories, 6.1g protein, 15g carbohydrates, 13.4g fat, 6.4g fiber, 13mg cholesterol, 88mg sodium, 811mg potassium

Avocado, Tomato and Olives Salad

Preparation time: 5 minutes

Cooking time: 0 minutes

Servings: 4

Ingredients:

- 2 tablespoons olive oil
- 2 avocados, peeled, pitted and cut into wedges
- 1 cup kalamata olives, pitted and halved
- 1 cup tomatoes, cubed
- 1 tablespoon ginger, grated
- A pinch of black pepper
- 2 cups baby arugula
- 1 tablespoon balsamic vinegar

Directions:

1. In a bowl, combine the avocados with the kalamata and the other ingredients, toss and serve as a side dish.

Nutrition info per serving: 320 calories, 3g protein, 13.9g carbohydrates, 30.4g fat, 8.7g fiber, 0mg cholesterol, 305mg sodium, 655mg potassium

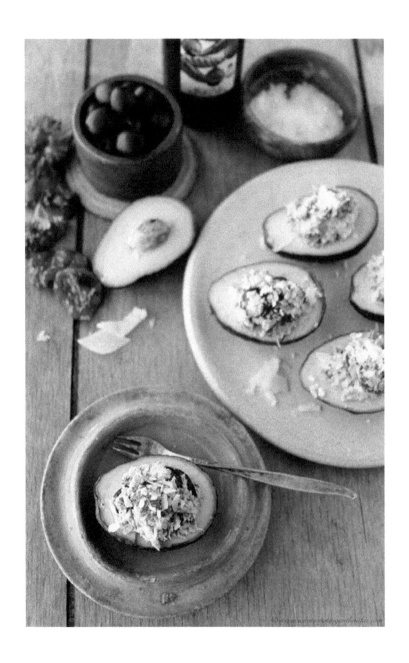

Radish and Olives Salad

Preparation time: 5 minutes

Cooking time: 0 minutes

Servings: 4

Ingredients:

- 2 green onions, sliced
- 1 pound radishes, cubed
- 2 tablespoons balsamic vinegar
- 2 tablespoon olive oil
- 1 teaspoon chili powder
- 1 cup black olives, pitted and halved
- A pinch of black pepper

Directions:

1. In a large salad bowl, combine radishes with the onions and the other ingredients, toss and serve as a side dish.

Nutrition info per serving: 123 calories, 1.3g protein, 6.9g carbohydrates, 10.8g fat, 3.3g fiber, 0mg cholesterol, 345mg sodium, 306mg potassium

Spinach and Endives Salad

Preparation time: 5 minutes

Cooking time: 0 minutes

Servings: 4

Ingredients:

- 2 endives, roughly shredded
- 1 tablespoon dill, chopped
- ¼ cup lemon juice
- ¼ cup olive oil
- 2 cups baby spinach
- 2 tomatoes, cubed
- 1 cucumber, sliced
- ½ cups walnuts, chopped

Directions:

1. In a large bowl, combine the endives with the spinach and the other ingredients, toss and serve as a side dish.

Nutrition info per serving: 238 calories, 5.7g protein, 8.4g carbohydrates, 22.3g fat, 3.1g fiber, 0mg cholesterol, 24mg sodium, 506mg potassium

Basil Olives Mix

Preparation time: 5 minutes

Cooking time: 0 minutes

Servings: 4

Ingredients:

- 2 tablespoons olive oil
- 1 tablespoon balsamic vinegar
- A pinch of black pepper
- 4 cups corn
- 2 cups black olives, pitted and halved
- 1 red onion, chopped
- ½ cup cherry tomatoes, halved
- 1 tablespoon basil, chopped
- 1 tablespoon jalapeno, chopped
- 2 cups romaine lettuce, shredded

Directions:

1. In a large bowl, combine the corn with the olives, lettuce and the other ingredients, toss well, divide between plates and serve as a side dish.

Nutrition info per serving: 290 calories, 6.2g protein, 37.6g carbohydrates, 16.1g fat, 7.4g fiber, 0mg cholesterol, 613mg sodium, 562mg potassium

Arugula Salad

Preparation time: 5 minutes

Cooking time: 0 minutes

Servings: 4

Ingredients:

- ¼ cup pomegranate seeds
- 5 cups baby arugula
- 6 tablespoons green onions, chopped
- 1 tablespoon balsamic vinegar
- 2 tablespoons olive oil
- 3 tablespoons pine nuts
- ½ shallot, chopped

Directions:

1. In a salad bowl, combine the arugula with the pomegranate and the other ingredients, toss and serve.

Nutrition info per serving: 120 calories, 1.8g protein, 4.2g carbohydrates, 11.6g fat, 0.9g fiber, 0mg cholesterol, 9mg sodium, 163mg potassium

Lemon Spinach

Preparation time: 10 minutes

Cooking time: 0 minutes

Servings: 4

Ingredients:

- 2 tablespoons olive oil
- 2 avocados, peeled, pitted and cut into wedges
- 3 cups baby spinach
- ¼ cup almonds, toasted and chopped
- 1 tablespoon lemon juice
- 1 tablespoon cilantro, chopped

Directions:

1. In a bowl, combine the avocados with the almonds, spinach and the other ingredients, toss and serve as a side dish.

Nutrition info per serving: 306 calories, 3.9g protein, 10.8g carbohydrates, 29.7g fat, 8g fiber, 0mg cholesterol, 25mg sodium, 663mg potassium

Green Beans Salad

Preparation time: 4 minutes

Cooking time: 0 minutes

Servings: 4

Ingredients:

- Juice of 1 lime
- 2 cups romaine lettuce, shredded
- 1 cup corn
- ½ pound green beans, blanched and halved
- 1 cucumber, chopped
- 1/3 cup chives, chopped

Directions:

1. In a bowl, combine the green beans with the corn and the other ingredients, toss and serve.

Nutrition info per serving: 67 calories, 3g protein, 15g carbohydrates, 0.7g fat, 3.6g fiber, 0mg cholesterol, 12mg sodium, 384mg potassium

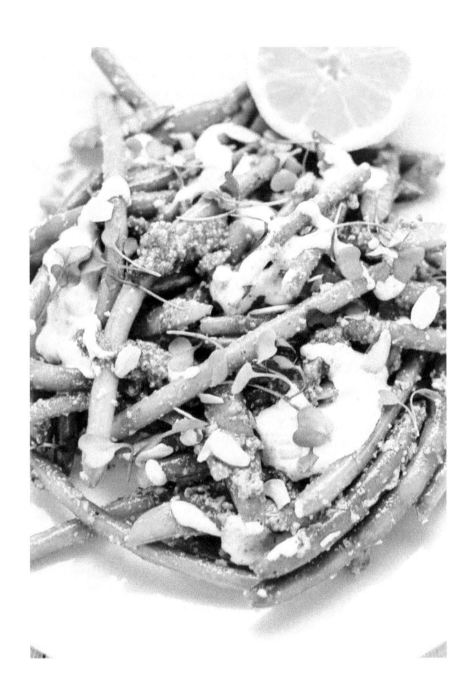

Endives Salad

Preparation time: 4 minutes

Cooking time: 0 minutes

Servings: 4

Ingredients:

- 3 tablespoons olive oil
- 2 endives, trimmed and shredded
- 2 tablespoons lime juice
- 1 tablespoon lime zest, grated
- 1 red onion, sliced
- 1 tablespoon balsamic vinegar
- 1 pound kale, torn
- A pinch of black pepper

Directions:

1. In a bowl, combine the endives with the kale and the other ingredients, toss well and serve cold as a side salad.

Nutrition info per serving: 160 calories, 3.9g protein, 15.1g carbohydrates, 10.6g fat, 2.8g fiber, 0mg cholesterol, 53mg sodium, 641mg potassium

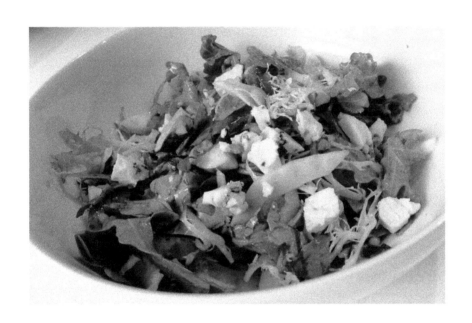

Chives Edamame Salad

Preparation time: 5 minutes

Cooking time: 6 minutes

Servings: 4

Ingredients:

- 2 tablespoons olive oil
- 2 tablespoons balsamic vinegar
- 2 garlic cloves, minced
- 3 cups edamame, shelled
- 1 tablespoon chives, chopped
- 2 shallots, chopped

Directions:

1. Heat up a pan with the oil over medium heat, add the edamame, the garlic and the other ingredients, toss, cook for 6 minutes, divide between plates and serve.

Nutrition info per serving: 350 calories, 25.1g protein, 22.7g carbohydrates, 20.1g fat, 8.1g fiber, 0mg cholesterol, 30mg sodium, 1221mg potassium

Grapes and Cucumber Salad

Preparation time: 5 minutes

Cooking time: 0 minutes

Servings: 4

Ingredients:

- 2 cups baby spinach
- 2 avocados, peeled, pitted and roughly cubed
- 1 cucumber, sliced
- 1 and ½ cups green grapes, halved
- 2 tablespoons avocado oil
- 1 tablespoon cider vinegar
- 2 tablespoons parsley, chopped
- A pinch of black pepper

Directions:

1. In a salad bowl, combine the baby spinach with the avocados and the other ingredients, toss and serve.

Nutrition info per serving: 274 calories, 3.1g protein, 18g carbohydrates, 23.4g fat, 7.8g fiber, 0mg cholesterol, 21mg sodium, 761mg potassium

Parmesan Eggplant Mix

Preparation time: 10 minutes

Cooking time: 20 minutes

Servings: 4

Ingredients:

- 2 big eggplants, roughly cubed
- 1 tablespoon oregano, chopped
- ½ cup low-fat parmesan, grated
- ¼ teaspoon garlic powder
- 2 tablespoons olive oil
- A pinch of black pepper

Directions:

1. In a baking pan combine the eggplants with the oregano and the other ingredients except the cheese and toss.
2. Sprinkle parmesan on top, introduce in the oven and bake at 370 degrees F for 20 minutes.
3. Divide between plates and serve as a side dish.

Nutrition info per serving: 154 calories, 4.9g protein, 14.5g carbohydrates, 10g fat, 8.6g fiber, 11mg cholesterol, 196mg sodium, 561mg potassium

Garlic Tomatoes Mix

Preparation time: 10 minutes

Cooking time: 20 minutes

Servings: 4

Ingredients:

- 2 pounds tomatoes, halved
- 1 tablespoon basil, chopped
- 3 tablespoons olive oil
- Zest of 1 lemon, grated
- 3 garlic cloves, minced
- ¼ cup low-fat parmesan, grated
- A pinch of black pepper

Directions:

1. In a baking pan, combine the tomatoes with the basil and the other ingredients except the cheese and toss.
2. Sprinkle the parmesan on top, introduce in the oven at 375 degrees F for 20 minutes, divide between plates and serve as a side dish.

Nutrition info per serving: 136 calories, 2.3g protein, 10g carbohydrates, 11g fat, 2.9g fiber, 0mg cholesterol, 20mg sodium, 553mg potassium

Turkey and Carrots Soup

Preparation time: 10 minutes

Cooking time: 25 minutes

Servings: 4

Ingredients:

- 1 pound chicken breast, skinless, boneless and cubed
- 2 cups cauliflower florets
- 1 tablespoon olive oil
- 1 red onion, chopped
- 1 tablespoon balsamic vinegar
- ½ cup red bell pepper, chopped
- A pinch of black pepper
- 2 garlic cloves, minced
- ½ cup low-sodium chicken stock
- 1 cup canned tomatoes, no-salt-added, chopped

Directions:

1. Heat up a pan with the oil over medium-high heat, add the onion, garlic and the meat and brown for 5 minutes.

2. Add the rest of the ingredients, toss and cook over medium heat for 20 minutes.
3. Divide everything into bowls and serve for lunch.

Nutrition info per serving: 200 calories, 26g protein, 8.7g carbohydrates, 6.6g fat, 2.6g fiber, 73mg cholesterol, 94mg sodium, 755mg potassium

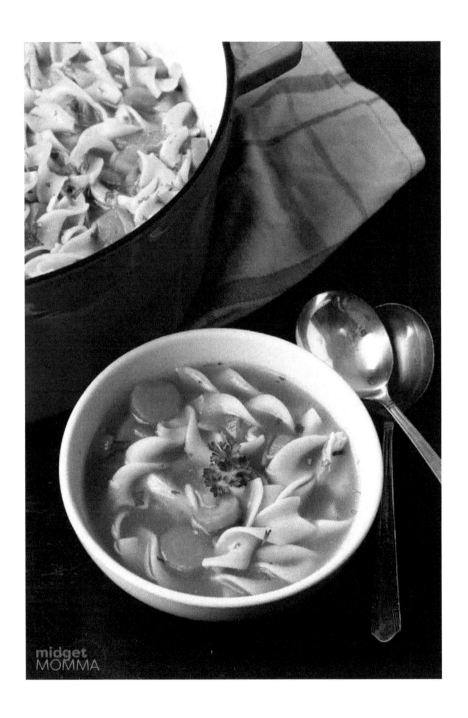

Tomato Soup

Preparation time: 10 minutes

Cooking time: 20 minutes

Servings: 4

Ingredients:

- 3 garlic cloves, minced
- 1 yellow onion, chopped
- 3 carrots, chopped
- 1 tablespoon olive oil
- 20 ounces roasted tomatoes, no-salt-added
- 2 cup low-sodium vegetable stock
- 1 tablespoon basil, dried
- 1 cup coconut cream
- A pinch of black pepper

Directions:

1. Heat up a pot with the oil over medium heat, add the onion and the garlic and sauté for 5 minutes.
2. Add the rest of the ingredients, stir, bring to a simmer, cook for 15 minutes, blend the soup using an immersion blender, divide into bowls and serve for lunch.

Nutrition info per serving: 241 calories, 3.3g protein, 18.6g carbohydrates, 17.8g fat, 4.2g fiber, 0mg cholesterol, 253mg sodium, 355mg potassium

Pork and Potatoes

Preparation time: 10 minutes

Cooking time: 30 minutes

Servings: 4

Ingredients:

- 4 pork chops, boneless
- 1 pound sweet potatoes, peeled and cut into wedges
- 1 tablespoon olive oil
- 1 cup vegetable stock, low-sodium
- A pinch of black pepper
- 1 teaspoon oregano, dried
- 1 teaspoon rosemary, dried
- 1 teaspoon basil, dried

Directions:

1. Heat up a pan with the oil over medium-high heat, add the pork chops and cook them for 4 minutes on each side.
2. Add the sweet potatoes and the rest of the ingredients, put the lid on and cook over medium heat for 20 minutes more stirring from time to time.

3. Divide everything between plates and serve.

Nutrition info per serving: 426 calories, 19.8g protein, 33.1g carbohydrates, 23.7g fat, 4.9g fiber, 69mg cholesterol, 164mg sodium, 1210mg potassium

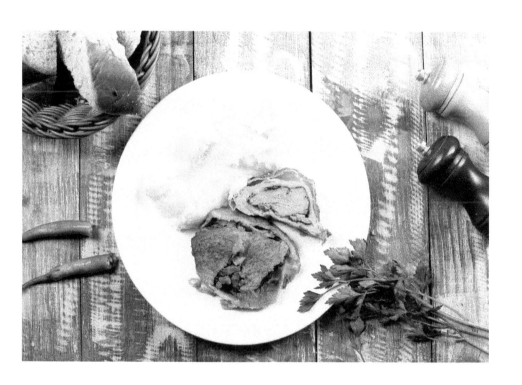

Trout Soup

Preparation time: 10 minutes

Cooking time: 25 minutes

Servings: 4

Ingredients:

- 1 yellow onion, chopped
- 12 cups low-sodium fish stock
- 1 pound carrots, sliced
- 1 pound trout fillets, boneless, skinless and cubed
- 1 tablespoon sweet paprika
- 1 cup tomatoes, cubed
- 1 tablespoon olive oil
- Black pepper to the taste

Directions:

1. Heat up a pot with the oil over medium-high heat, add the onion, stir and sauté for 5 minutes.
2. Add the fish, carrots and the rest of the ingredients, bring to a simmer and cook over medium heat for 20 minutes.

3. Ladle the soup into bowls and serve.

Nutrition info per serving: 31 c6alories, 32.1g protein, 16.4g carbohydrates, 13.4g fat, 4.6g fiber, 84mg cholesterol, 158mg sodium, 1075mg potassium

Garlic Turkey Stew

Preparation time: 10 minutes

Cooking time: 45 minutes

Servings: 4

Ingredients:

- 1 turkey breast, skinless, boneless and cubed
- 2 fennel bulbs, sliced
- 1 tablespoon olive oil
- 2 bay leaves
- 1 yellow onion, chopped
- 1 cup canned tomatoes, no-salt-added
- 2 low-sodium beef stock
- 3 garlic cloves, chopped
- Black pepper to the taste

Directions:

1. Heat up a pan with the oil over medium heat, add the onion and the meat and brown for 5 minutes.
2. Add the fennel and the rest of the ingredients, bring to a simmer and cook

over medium heat for 40 minutes, stirring from time to time.

3. Divide the stew into bowls and serve.

Nutrition info per serving: 96 c6alories, 3.4g protein, 14g carbohydrates, 3.9g fat, 4.9g fiber, 0mg cholesterol, 137mg sodium, 644mg potassium

Tomato Eggplant Soup

Preparation time: 10 minutes

Cooking time: 30 minutes

Servings: 4

Ingredients:

- 2 big eggplants, roughly cubed
- 1 quart low-sodium vegetable stock
- 2 tablespoons no-salt-added tomato paste
- 1 red onion, chopped
- 1 tablespoon olive oil
- 1 tablespoon cilantro, chopped
- A pinch of black pepper

Directions:

1. Heat up a pot with the oil over medium heat, add the onion, stir and sauté for 5 minutes.
2. Add the eggplants and the other ingredients, bring to a simmer over medium heat, cook for 25 minutes, divide into bowls and serve.

Nutrition info per serving: 102 c6alories, 3g protein, 16.2g carbohydrates, 3.8g fat, 6.8g fiber, 0mg cholesterol, 152mg sodium, 566mg potassium

Potatoes Soup

Preparation time: 10 minutes

Cooking time: 25 minutes

Servings: 4

Ingredients:

- 4 cups veggie stock
- 2 tablespoons avocado oil
- 2 sweet potatoes, peeled and cubed
- 2 yellow onions, chopped
- 2 garlic cloves, minced
- 1 cup coconut milk
- A pinch of black pepper
- ½ teaspoon basil, chopped

Directions:

1. Heat up a pot with the oil over medium heat, add the onion and the garlic, stir and sauté for 5 minutes.
2. Add the sweet potatoes and the rest of the ingredients, bring to a simmer and cook over medium heat for 20 minutes.
3. Blend the soup using an immersion blender, ladle into bowls and serve for lunch.

Nutrition info per serving: 236 calories, 3.7g protein, 23.8g carbohydrates, 15.3g fat, 5.4g fiber, 0mg cholesterol, 155mg sodium, 703mg potassium

Chili Chicken Soup

Preparation time: 10 minutes

Cooking time: 30 minutes

Servings: 4

Ingredients:

- 1 quart veggie stock, low-sodium
- 1 tablespoon ginger, grated
- 1 yellow onion, chopped
- 1 tablespoon olive oil
- 1 pound chicken breast, skinless, boneless and cubed
- ½ pound white mushrooms, sliced
- 4 Thai chilies, chopped
- ¼ cup lime juice
- ¼ cup cilantro, chopped
- A pinch of black pepper

Directions:

1. Heat up a pot with the oil over medium heat, add the onion, ginger, chilies and the meat, stir and brown for 5 minutes.
2. Add the mushrooms, stir and cook for 5 minutes more.

3. Add the rest of the ingredients, bring to a simmer and cook over medium heat for 20 minutes more.
4. Ladle the soup into bowls and serve right away.

Nutrition info per serving: 197 calories, 26.5g protein, 7.4g carbohydrates, 6.6g fat, 1.6g fiber, 73mg cholesterol, 173mg sodium, 696mg potassium

Salmon Skillet

Preparation time: 10 minutes

Cooking time: 20 minutes

Servings: 4

Ingredients:

- 4 salmon fillet, boneless
- 3 garlic cloves, minced
- 1 yellow onion, chopped
- Black pepper to the taste
- 2 tablespoons olive oil
- Juice of 1 lime
- 1 tablespoon lime zest, grated
- 1 tablespoon thyme, chopped

Directions:

1. Heat up a pan with the oil over medium-high heat, add the onion and garlic, stir and sauté for 5 minutes.
2. Add the fish and cook it for 3 minutes on each side.
3. Add the rest of the ingredients, cook everything for 10 minutes more, divide between plates and serve for lunch.

Nutrition info per serving: 253 calories, 35.1g protein, 4.1g carbohydrates, 11.1g fat, 1.1g fiber, 78mg cholesterol, 80mg sodium, 741mg potassium

Potato and Spinach Salad

Preparation time: 10 minutes

Cooking time: 20 minutes

Servings: 4

Ingredients:

- 2 tomatoes, chopped
- 2 avocados, pitted and chopped
- 2 cups baby spinach
- 2 scallions, chopped
- 1 pound gold potatoes, boiled, peeled and cut into wedges
- 1 tablespoon olive oil
- 1 tablespoon lemon juice
- 1 yellow onion, chopped
- 2 garlic cloves, minced
- Black pepper to the taste
- 1 bunch cilantro, chopped

Directions:

1. Heat up a pan with the oil over medium-high heat, add the onion, scallions and the garlic, stir and sauté for 5 minutes.

2. Add the potatoes, toss gently and cook for 5 minutes more.
3. Add the rest of the ingredients, toss, cook over medium heat for 10 minutes more, divide into bowls and serve for lunch.

Nutrition info per serving: 342 calories, 5g protein, 33.5g carbohydrates, 23.4g fat, 11.7g fiber, 0mg cholesterol, 25mg sodium, 1262mg potassium

Ground Beef Skillet

Preparation time: 10 minutes

Cooking time: 20 minutes

Servings: 4

Ingredients:

- 1 pound beef, ground
- 1 red onion, chopped
- 1 tablespoon olive oil
- 1 cup cherry tomatoes, halved
- ½ red bell pepper, chopped
- Black pepper to the taste
- 1 tablespoon chives, chopped
- 1 tablespoon rosemary, chopped
- 3 tablespoons low-sodium beef stock

Directions:

1. Heat up a pan with the oil over medium heat, add the onion and the bell pepper, stir and sauté for 5 minutes.
2. Add the meat, stir and brown it for another 5 minutes.

3. Add the rest of the ingredients, toss, cook for 10 minutes, divide into bowls and serve for lunch.

Nutrition info per serving: 265 calories, 35.3g protein, 5.5g carbohydrates, 10.7g fat, 1.4g fiber, 101mg cholesterol, 85mg sodium, 634mg potassium

Shrimp and Arugula Salad

Preparation time: 5 minutes

Cooking time: 0 minutes

Servings: 4

Ingredients:

- 1 orange, peeled and cut into segments
- 1 pound shrimp, cooked, peeled and deveined
- 2 cups baby arugula
- 1 avocado, pitted, peeled and cubed
- 2 tablespoons olive oil
- 2 tablespoons balsamic vinegar
- Juice of½ orange
- Salt and black pepper

Directions:

1. In a salad bowl, mix combine the shrimp with the oranges and the other ingredients, toss and serve for lunch.

Nutrition info per serving: 323 calories, 27.5g protein, 11.9g carbohydrates, 18.9g fat, 4.6g fiber,

239mg cholesterol, 283mg sodium, 561mg potassium

Coconut Broccoli Cream

Preparation time: 10 minutes

Cooking time: 40 minutes

Servings: 4

Ingredients:

- 2 pounds broccoli florets
- 1 yellow onion, chopped
- 1 tablespoon olive oil
- Black pepper to the taste
- 2 garlic cloves, minced
- 3 cups low-sodium beef stock
- 1 cup coconut milk
- 2 tablespoons cilantro, chopped

Directions:

1. Heat up a pot with the oil over medium heat, add the onion and the garlic, stir and sauté for 5 minutes.
2. Add the broccoli and the other ingredients except the coconut milk, bring to a simmer and cook over medium heat for 35 minutes more.

3. Blend the soup using an immersion blender, add the coconut milk, pulse again, divide into bowls and serve.

Nutrition info per serving: 275 calories, 12.5g protein, 21g carbohydrates, 18.6g fat, 7.8g fiber, 0mg cholesterol, 648mg sodium, 918mg potassium

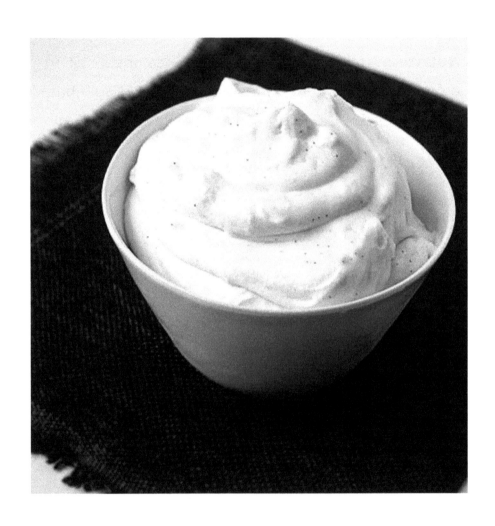

Cabbage and Leek Soup

Preparation time: 10 minutes

Cooking time: 40 minutes

Servings: 4

Ingredients:

- 1 big green cabbage head, roughly shredded
- 1 yellow onion, chopped
- 1 tablespoon olive oil
- Black pepper to the taste
- 1 leek, chopped
- 2 cups canned tomatoes, low-sodium
- 4 cups chicken stock, low-sodium
- 1 tablespoon cilantro, chopped

Directions:

1. Heat up a pot with the oil over medium heat, add the onion and the leek, stir and cook for 5 minutes.
2. Add the cabbage and the rest of the ingredients except the cilantro, bring to a simmer and cook over medium heat for 35 minutes.

3. Ladle the soup into bowls, sprinkle the cilantro on top and serve.

Nutrition info per serving: 125 calories, 4.4g protein, 20.3g carbohydrates, 4.5g fat, 6.5g fiber, 0mg cholesterol, 806mg sodium, 613mg potassium

Dill Cauliflower Soup

Preparation time: 10 minutes

Cooking time: 40 minutes

Servings: 4

Ingredients:

- 2 pounds cauliflower florets
- 1 red onion, chopped
- 1 tablespoon olive oil
- 1 cup tomato puree, low sodium
- Black pepper to the taste
- 1 cup celery, chopped
- 6 cups low-sodium chicken stock
- 1 tablespoon dill, chopped

Directions:

1. Heat up a pot with the oil over medium-high heat, add the onion and the celery, stir and sauté for 5 minutes.
2. Add the cauliflower and the rest of the ingredients, bring to a simmer and cook over medium heat for 35 minutes more.
3. Divide the soup into bowls and serve.

Nutrition info per serving: 150 calories, 9.5g protein, 22.4g carbohydrates, 3.9g fat, 7.6g fiber, 0mg cholesterol, 211mg sodium, 1028mg potassium

Parsley Pork Soup

Preparation time: 10 minutes

Cooking time: 40 minutes

Servings: 4

Ingredients:

- 1 pound pork stew meat, cubed
- Black pepper to the taste
- 5 leeks, chopped
- 1 yellow onion, chopped
- 2 tablespoons olive oil
- 1 tablespoon parsley, chopped
- 6 cups low-sodium beef stock

Directions:

1. Heat up a pot with the oil over medium-high heat, add the onion and the leeks, stir and sauté for 5 minutes.
2. Add the meat, stir and brown for 5 minutes more.
3. Add the rest of the ingredients, bring to a simmer and cook over medium heat for 30 minutes.
4. Ladle the soup into bowls and serve.

Nutrition info per serving: 402 calories, 41.2g protein, 18.4g carbohydrates, 18.3g fat, 2.6g fiber, 98mg cholesterol, 766mg sodium, 671mg potassium

Minty Shrimp and Olives Salad

Preparation time: 5 minutes

Cooking time: 20 minutes

Servings: 4

Ingredients:

- 1/3 cup low-sodium vegetable stock
- 2 tablespoons olive oil
- 2 cups broccoli florets
- 1 pound shrimp, peeled and deveined
- Black pepper to the taste
- 1 yellow onion, chopped
- 4 cherry tomatoes, halved
- 2 garlic cloves, minced
- Juice of ½ lemon
- ½ cup kalamata olives, pitted and cut into halves
- 1 tablespoon mint, chopped

Directions:

1. Heat up a pan with the oil over medium-high heat, add the onion and the garlic, stir and sauté for 3 minutes.
2. Add the shrimp, toss and cook for 2 minutes more.
3. Add the broccoli and the other ingredients, toss, cook everything for 10 minutes, divide into bowls and serve for lunch.

Nutrition info per serving: 267 calories, 28.9g protein, 13.8g carbohydrates, 11.2g fat, 3.9g fiber, 239mg cholesterol, 452mg sodium, 682mg potassium

Shrimp Soup

Preparation time: 10 minutes

Cooking time: 20 minutes

Servings: 4

Ingredients:

- 1 quart low-sodium chicken stock
- ½ pound shrimp, peeled and deveined
- ½ pound cod fillets, boneless, skinless and cubed
- 2 tablespoons olive oil
- 2 teaspoons chili powder
- 1 teaspoon sweet paprika
- 2 shallots, chopped
- A pinch of black pepper
- 1 tablespoon dill, chopped

Directions:

1. Heat up a pot with the oil over medium heat, add the shallots, stir and sauté for 5 minutes.
2. Add the shrimp and the cod, and cook for 5 minutes more.

3. Add the rest of the ingredients, bring to a simmer and cook over medium heat for 10 minutes.
4. Divide the soup into bowls and serve.

Nutrition info per serving: 190 calories, 24.8g protein, 3.2g carbohydrates, 8.8g fat, 0.8g fiber, 147mg cholesterol, 358mg sodium, 176mg potassium

Balsamic Shrimp

Preparation time: 10 minutes

Cooking time: 10 minutes

Servings: 4

Ingredients:

- 2 pounds shrimp, peeled and deveined
- 1 cup cherry tomatoes, halved
- 1 tablespoon olive oil
- 4 green onion, chopped
- 1 tablespoon balsamic vinegar
- 1 tablespoon chives, chopped

Directions:

1. Heat up a pan with the oil over medium heat, add the onion, and the cherry tomatoes, stir and sauté for 4 minutes.
2. Add the shrimp and the other ingredients, cook for 6 minutes more, divide between plates and serve.

Nutrition info per serving: 313 calories, 52.4g protein, 6.4g carbohydrates, 7.5g fat, 1g fiber,

478mg cholesterol, 558mg sodium, 537mg potassium

Spinach and Tomato Stew

Preparation time: 10 minutes

Cooking time: 15 minutes

Servings: 4

Ingredients:

- 1 tablespoons olive oil
- 1 teaspoon ginger, grated
- 2 garlic cloves, minced
- 1 yellow onion, chopped
- 2 tomatoes, chopped
- 1 cup canned tomatoes, no-salt-added
- 1 teaspoon cumin, ground
- A pinch of black pepper
- 1 cup low-sodium vegetable stock
- 2 pounds spinach leaves

Directions:

1. Heat up a pot with the oil over medium heat, add the ginger, garlic and the onion, stir and sauté for 5 minutes.
2. Add the tomatoes, canned tomatoes and the other ingredients, toss gently, bring to a simmer and cook for 10 minutes more.

3. Divide the stew into bowls and serve.

Nutrition info per serving: 120 calories, 8.1g protein, 14.5g carbohydrates, 4.7g fat, 6.5g fiber, 0mg cholesterol, 207mg sodium, 1473mg potassium

Cilantro Peppers and Cauliflower Mix

Preparation time: 10 minutes

Cooking time: 25 minutes

Servings: 4

Ingredients:

- 1 red onion, chopped
- 1 tablespoon olive oil
- 2 garlic cloves, minced
- 1 red bell pepper, chopped
- 1 green bell pepper, chopped
- 1 tablespoon lime juice
- 1 pound cauliflower florets
- 14 ounces canned tomatoes, chopped, low sodium
- 2 teaspoons curry powder
- A pinch of black pepper
- 2 cups coconut cream
- 1 tablespoon cilantro, chopped

Directions:

1. Heat up a pot with the oil over medium heat, add the onion and the garlic, stir and cook for 5 minutes.
2. Add the bell peppers and the other ingredients, bring everything to a simmer and cook over medium heat for 20 minutes.
3. Divide everything into bowls and serve.

Nutrition info per serving: 384 calories, 7g protein, 23.8g carbohydrates, 32.7g fat, 8.5g fiber, 0mg cholesterol, 60mg sodium, 1065mg potassium

Rosemary Carrot Stew

Preparation time: 10 minutes

Cooking time: 30 minutes

Servings: 4

Ingredients:

- 1 yellow onion, chopped
- 2 tablespoons olive oil
- 2 garlic cloves, minced
- 4 zucchinis, sliced
- 2 carrots, sliced
- 1 teaspoon sweet paprika
- ¼ teaspoon chili powder
- A pinch of black pepper
- ½ cup tomatoes, chopped
- 2 cups low-sodium vegetable stock
- 1 tablespoon chives, chopped
- 1 tablespoon rosemary, chopped

Directions:

1. Heat up a pot with the oil over medium heat, add the onion and the garlic, stir and sauté for 5 minutes.

2. Add the zucchinis, carrots and the other ingredients, bring to a simmer and cook for 25 minutes more.
3. Divide the stew in to bowls and serve right away for lunch.

Nutrition info per serving: 134 calories, 4.4g protein, 15g carbohydrates, 7.7g fat, 4.4g fiber, 0mg cholesterol, 80mg sodium, 737mg potassium

Cabbage Stew

Preparation time: 10 minutes

Cooking time: 25 minutes

Servings: 4

Ingredients:

- 2 tablespoons olive oil
- 1 red cabbage head, shredded
- 1 red onion, chopped
- 1 pound green beans, trimmed and halved
- 2 garlic cloves, minced
- 7 ounces canned tomatoes, no-salt-added chopped
- 2 cups low-sodium vegetable stock
- A pinch of black pepper
- 1 tablespoon dill, chopped

Directions:

1. Heat up a pot with the oil, over medium heat, add the onion and the garlic, stir and sauté for 5 minutes.
2. Add the cabbage and the other ingredients, stir, cover and simmer over medium heat for 20 minutes.

3. Divide into bowls and serve for lunch.

Nutrition info per serving: 171 calories, 6.3g protein, 24.4g carbohydrates, 7.5g fat, 9.7g fiber, 0mg cholesterol, 79mg sodium, 730mg potassium

Mushroom Soup

Preparation time: 5 minutes

Cooking time: 30 minutes

Servings: 4

Ingredients:

- 1 yellow onion, chopped
- 1 tablespoon olive oil
- 1 red chili pepper, chopped
- 1 teaspoon chili powder
- ½ teaspoon hot paprika
- 4 garlic cloves, minced
- 1 pound white mushrooms, sliced
- 6 cups low-sodium vegetable stock
- 1 cup tomatoes, chopped
- ½ tablespoon parsley, chopped

Directions:

1. Heat up a pot with the oil, over medium heat, add the onion, chili pepper, hot paprika, chili powder and the garlic, stir and sauté for 5 minutes.
2. Add the mushrooms, stir and cook for 5 minutes more.

3. Add the rest of the ingredients, bring to a simmer and cook over medium heat for 20 minutes.
4. Divide the soup into bowls and serve.

Nutrition info per serving: 103 calories, 7.5g protein, 11g carbohydrates, 4.1g fat, 2.6g fiber, 0mg cholesterol, 122mg sodium, 537mg potassium

Oregano Pork

Preparation time: 10 minutes

Cooking time: 30 minutes

Servings: 4

Ingredients:

- 2 pounds pork stew meat, cubed
- 2 tablespoons chili paste
- 1 yellow onion, chopped
- 2 garlic cloves, minced
- 1 tablespoon olive oil
- 2 cups low-sodium beef stock
- 1 tablespoon oregano, chopped

Directions:

1. Heat up a pot with the oil, over medium-high heat, add the onion and the garlic, stir and sauté for 5 minutes.
2. Add the meat and brown it for 5 minutes more.
3. Add the rest of the ingredients, bring to a simmer and cook over medium heat for 20 minutes more.
4. Divide the mix into bowls and serve.

Nutrition info per serving: 565 calories, 69.4g protein, 7.8g carbohydrates, 26.8g fat, 1.1g fiber, 198mg cholesterol, 475mg sodium, 916mg potassium

Lightning Source UK Ltd.
Milton Keynes UK
UKHW020824170621
385666UK00005B/125